FROM OUR ARMS TO HIS

FROM OUR ARMS TO HIS

A Caregiver's Journey of Love, Faith, and Frustration

Dianne Codding Horncastle

2024

To care for those who once cared for us is one of the highest honors
Tia Walker

Copyright © 2024 Dianne Codding Horncastle All rights reserved.

No part of this book may be reproduced, stored in a retrieval system, or transmitted in any form or by any means, electronic, mechanical, photocopying, recording, or otherwise, without express written permission of the publisher.

ISBN: 9798336750669

Imprint: Independently published

Cover design by: Dianne Codding Horncastle

Printed in the United States of America

Scripture quotations marked (NIV) are taken from the Holy Bible, New International Version®, NIV®. Copyright © 1973, 1978, 1984, 2011 by Biblica, Inc.™ Used by permission of Zondervan. All rights reserved worldwide. www.zondervan.comThe "NIV" and "New International Version" are trademarks registered in the United States Patent and Trademark Office by Biblica, Inc.™

Scripture quotations marked NLT are taken from the Holy Bible, New Living Translation, Copyright © 1996, 2004, 2015 by Tyndale House Foundation. Used by permission of Tyndale House Publishers, Inc., Carol Stream, Illinois 60188. All rights reserved.

Scripture quotations marked (TLB) are taken from The Living Bible, copyright © 1971. Used by permission of Tyndale House Publishers, Carol Stream, Illinois 60188. All rights reserved.

"New Revised Standard Version Bible, copyright 1989, Division of Christian Education of the National Council of the Churches of Christ in the United States of America. Used by permission. All rights reserved."

Dedication

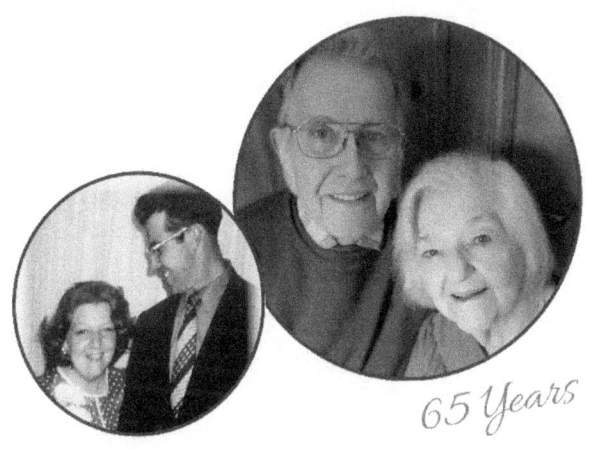

65 Years

In many pictures, over the years, my dad is looking and smiling at my mom. When I asked him about it, he said, "I just couldn't believe that such a beautiful woman was mine."

To Mom & Dad, my first true loves.
Who were not perfect but were
God's perfect gift to me.

The Love of a Family is Life's Richest Blessing

Acknowledgment

I am profoundly grateful to my husband, partner, and best friend, Kelly, who selflessly gave up vacations and holidays together while I spent all my available time in New York.

My favorite activities include sharing writing ideas and brainstorming with you over coffee or a margarita. Your diligent biblical research added depth and support to the themes woven throughout these pages.

Your unwavering encouragement during moments of doubt and openness to exploring innovative ideas helped shape and refine this work. Thank you for being a constant source of inspiration and wisdom, always reminding me that my words are a gift from God meant to be shared. This book would not have been the same without your support and encouragement.

Thank you, thank you, thank you…With all my love,

"I have found the one whom my soul loves." Dianne

CONTENTS

HOW TO USE THIS BOOK _____ 1

PREFACE _____ 3

INTRODUCTION _____ 5

PRAY TOGETHER _____ 9

THE FEAR IS REAL _____ 13

   Honesty Defuses Everything _____ 16

GOD'S PROMISES _____ 21

STANDING IN THE GAP _____ 23

THE WEARY CAREGIVER _____ 27

   Validate And Redirect _____ 32
   Creating Solutions _____ 37

CHERISHED MEMORIES _____ 43

   A Christmas to Remember _____ 46

THE GRAY AREA _____ 51

WORDS OF JOY _____ 57

TRANSITIONS _____ 61

   Walking In Their Shoes _____ 64
   I'll Think About That Tomorrow _____ 67
   There is Truth in The Gray Area _____ 71

THE RALLY	74
THE LAST GOODBYE	**77**
WHAT COMES NEXT	81
THE AFTERSHOCK	**85**
20-SECOND HUGS TO YOU	87
THE DISBELIEF OF LOSS	89
WE ARE BUT A BREATH A EULOGY	**91**
A CELEBRATION OF GOD'S GIFT	96
THE SAND CEREMONY	**99**
THANK YOU	**101**
REFERENCES	**103**
ABOUT THE AUTHOR	**105**

How to use this Book

This book is not designed like a traditional devotional but as a companion guide for caregivers navigating the twisting path of caring for a loved one. The chapters are intentionally short, each one introducing a subject meant to spark conversation and prayer among you and your loved one.

In my journey, devotions and prayer with my mom offered unique opportunities to share deeper conversations. After prayer came exercises that always began with "praise arms"—raising each arm as best we could and sharing what we were grateful for that morning.

The prayers and exercises are examples to offer a jumping-off point. I encourage you to make your prayers heartfelt, honest, and vulnerable, reflecting your unique journey.

While our stories may share similarities, they are not the same. Your circumstances and heartache are uniquely yours, making them more challenging in ways only you can fully understand. I hope you'll find enough commonality to discover laughter, solace, and solutions for what your journey brings.

Caregiving often calls us to lean into love we didn't know possible
Tia Walker

To be notified of additional writings by Dianne, please join the mailing list using the link below.

[JOIN - Dianne's Email List](#)

If you like what you read, a review on Kindle or Amazon would mean the world to me.

Preface

As a child, my mother and I did not share a best friend, you-are-my-world type relationship.

I was my mother's third child and one of six by the time I was four. She did not have time for a you-are-my-world relationship.

My childhood was happy, safe, and secure, but I often felt like my mom, and I were at odds with each other. I was a lot like her, (bossy, take-control, and perceptive) and although I was too young to understand, we frequently experienced a power struggle. I didn't believe my mom liked me very much.

I went to college out of state, married, and moved away at 21. Our relationship was happy, but there was little one-on-one bonding time.

In my early thirties, I moved home, my brother had just passed, and I took new stock in my life. I moved close to my parents, and it was during those years that we developed a deeper relationship.

As mothers and daughters, we built a girl's network called Yaya's. We spent long weekends together, sharing and caring for each other. In those moments, I saw a new depth to my mother, the woman, a person that I had never seen, and I loved it.

When you come from a large family, it is hard to have one-on-one relationship-building time; there is always someone else in the room.

In the last 6 months of my mom's life, I built a memory book of my parents' 65 years together. As I laid experience after experience down on paper, I began to discover the whole of the whole of a woman who loved God and gave her life to make other people happy the only way she knew how. I loved growing in this truth and realizing I was one of my mom's 'you-are-my-world' relationships.

My mother encouraged me to be her wings; to fly as she never dared to. ~ Unknown

---

Introduction

As I draft this small book, it has been one month since my mom passed gently into the arms of Jesus, and each passing moment is bitter-sweet. My memories are so full of joy while my heart is equally broken.

In this life, while one family celebrates, the next mourns; it is the ebb and flow of life. How blessed are we that we have loved and belonged to someone else so deeply that our hearts cannot comprehend a life without them?

It makes me reflect on God's love and how His heart must ache when even one child is lost. At that moment, the presence of another loved one offers no solace.

I incessantly prayed that I could be with my mother when she passed. The odds were against me, but God delivered beautifully, and I was holding my mom in my arms as she transitioned. I don't believe I will ever forget the pure love and intimacy I felt.

If you are traveling a similar path, we are kindred spirits, and I wish you many blessings of joy, peace, and resolve throughout the journey.

The Lord bless you and keep you; the Lord make his face shine on you and be gracious to you; the Lord turn his face toward you and give you peace.
~ Numbers 6:24-26 NIV

My mom was 90 years old (two weeks from 91) when she passed. Although she had some health issues, it was in the last nine months that she took a turn for the worse.

My Dad became her primary caregiver, and the initial challenge was getting her to eat; she was losing weight, her body was becoming frail, and her memory was faltering, but she continued to play cards daily and crack jokes right on point.

My four siblings lived locally and stepped up to fill the gaps and support my father.

I lived 1300 miles away with no reasonable way to help. I prayed regularly for God to show me how to be a part of the solution; it weighed heavy on my heart. I wanted to support my family, I knew God had prepared me for this, and I wanted to be with my mom,

My prayers were answered when the small nonprofit I worked for generously allowed me a 60-day opportunity to be with my family. My story starts here.

When a journey takes you to the deepest valleys of your soul, you discover hidden strength that elevates you to the highest mountain peaks, and the view changes you forever.

Pray Together

Although we are a family of faith, we have not been a family that prays together regularly until recently.

I learned to pray together with my husband. Initially, I let my husband pray for us, our needs, and our loved ones, but at some point, I realized my voice was equally important for several reasons.

- It is beautiful to hear our name used in prayer and to know that our loved one is petitioning God on our behalf. I wanted my husband to hear his name in my prayers.

- There is a sweet vulnerability and intimacy in heartfelt, tear-filled, raw prayers that enhance and deepen relationships.

- Words and feelings that are difficult to express to each other outside of prayer may be easier to share through prayers.

I call this allowing God to stand in the gap. We all fall short due to egos, emotions, past hurts, etc. In shared prayer, we honestly confess our shortcomings to God, seeking forgiveness and guidance. This reinforces our intentions and our need for grace with God and our prayer partner.

In the past few years, our family has faced serious medical diagnoses and lost loved ones. Regardless of whether it was comfortable, we needed to come together physically or virtually to pray for God's intervention. This allowed loved ones to hear their names lifted to God, share the fears in our hearts, and remind each other of God's power and love.

That new practice of praying together enriched my time with my mom. Our morning routine, after she was dressed, included devotions, shared reflections, gratitude, prayers, and exercise. These moments are ones I will cherish forever. We discussed our fears and feelings, growing closer every day.

I will share more about these experiences as we move through this book. I'm sharing this now to encourage you to consider the benefits of praying together and to get comfortable praying and sharing honest moments with your loved ones.

For where two or three gather in my name, there am I with them."
~ Matthew 18:20 NIV

Today, begin the bold journey of praying out loud together. At first, it might feel strange, intimidating, or even embarrassing, but remember, God sees your heart long before He hears your words.

When I started praying out loud, I felt embarrassed that my prayers weren't fluid or eloquent. But the more I prayed, the less those feelings held me back, and the blessings outweighed the initial discomfort.

Ask your loved one if you can pray together; I'm confident they will say yes. If they don't feel ready, kindly ask for a moment to pray alone, then spend those few minutes praying quietly aloud.

Start by asking God for confidence. It's honest and shows your vulnerability, allowing your loved one to hear your genuine trepidation. Invite God to gently guide both of you as you share this unknown journey of change, discomfort, daily devotions, and discovery of new opportunities to bless and be blessed. And of course, add any other heartfelt petitions to God.

Remember, keep your prayers simple, honest, and authentic.

The Fear Is Real

God tells us 365 times in the Bible to 'fear not' in one way or another. I have always considered that intentional; one for every day of the year.

Regardless of our faith, we still fear. We fear loss, pain, heartache, harm, danger, the unknown, and more. God created our bodies to naturally react with fear to alert and keep us safe from danger. But he also lovingly tells us to 'fear not' because He is bigger than the object of our fear.

Tell that to my racing heart.

In those precious days with my mom, fear would often overwhelm her, causing her eyes to fill with tears as she sobbed, struggling to catch her breath. Anxiety and sorrow would tighten her chest, leaving her gasping for air. During these times, we would breathe deeply together and pray for God's calming presence. Gradually, as we prayed, her body would begin to relax, and a sense of peace would gently replace the fear.

One day, while I was alone and not doing anything specific, I was suddenly consumed by a tightness in my throat and chest, unable to breathe and filled with tears. It lasted less than 30 seconds. I assume it was my body reacting physically to the reality that I would soon lose my mother. Regardless, the fear was crushing, and I had a new understanding of what my mom was experiencing.

The fear is real. As Christians, we may think that admitting to the fear is admitting to a lack of faith.

God walks with us in our fear. He gives us peace and enables us to expand our faith in those moments. And he forgives us for our inadequacy.

Peter, a close friend of Jesus who walked alongside Him for over three years, denied Him in a moment of fear. Fear is real, and we are all human. Yet, just as He did for Peter, Jesus stands in the gap between our faith and fear, offering us His amazing grace.

Honesty defuses everything. Talking about fear together may help to release the anxiety that surrounds the fear.

As you hold your loved one's hands today, take a moment to talk about fear. Share a genuine story of a time when you felt afraid and uncertain. You may even share how it shook or deepened your faith. Ask them if they've had a similar experience and give them time to share.

Pray together, thanking God for walking with you through this unknown journey and for the gift of waking up today to face another day together. Ask God to stand in the gap between your fear and your faith, helping you both to speak openly and honestly about your fears and anxieties.

Side note: When I prayed with my mom, I always focused on thanking God for the new day we were given, together. We have no promise of tomorrow, and I was deeply grateful to be by her side, facing this journey with her. I couldn't bring myself to thank God solely for Mom waking up each morning, knowing she was moving closer to death. Instead, I thanked Him for the gift of us waking up together, one more day at a time.

So do not fear, for I am with you; do not be dismayed, for I am your God. I will strengthen you and help you; I will uphold you with my righteous right hand.
~Isaiah 41:10 NIV

For I am the Lord your God who takes hold of your right hand and says to you, do not fear; I will help you.
~ Isaiah 41:13 NIV

Honesty Defuses Everything

For me, the fear of loss was not just about losing my mom; it was the fear of losing life as I knew it. The fear of losing traditional holidays, the fear of losing my friend, my yaya sister, the matriarch of our family, and the wife and partner of my dad. The fear that I might not breathe again.

Knowing that I had been so blessed to have both my parents to such an old age and that most people experience this same loss was not consoling. Somehow, I thought my situation was different. No one else had loved their mom this much, and no one else could understand the turmoil and upheaval I was feeling.

This is true, every relationship is between two people alone. Your relationship with your loved one is yours alone, unique to you and them; there is no one with the exact relationship.

Initially, I had not considered that my mom was experiencing the same fear and heartbreak. She would also lose the people she loved the most, a life well-built, and the man she had shared life with for 65 years.

My mom's fear went beyond a fear of loss. She was facing a new, unknown season—and a new kind of fear. Where I was losing one relationship, she was losing many relationships.

When my siblings and I started staying with Mom and Dad to help through the night, we purchased a baby monitor to ensure we could hear if my father needed help.

One evening after a recent doctor's visit, Mom tearfully clung to my father, sharing her fears. She said she had hardly urinated that day, and she was afraid her kidneys were shutting down. She asked my father why he wasn't upset since the doctor had just told them she had only weeks to live. My dad, unaware of this conversation with the doctor, tried to convince her otherwise, to no avail. She needed Dad to stay up with her and hold her.

Be strong and courageous. Do not be afraid; do not be discouraged, for the Lord your God will be with you wherever you go. ~Joshua 1:9 NIV

Do not be anxious about anything, but in every situation, by prayer and petition, with thanksgiving, present your requests to God. ~Philippians 4:6 NIV

This marked the beginning of many months of staying up with Mom late into the night. She refused to go to bed before midnight, complaining that she lay alone in the dark, waiting for the first light to come through the window. Her mind could not rest.

The next day, I reached out to the doctor to clarify. Although he did not recall having that conversation with my mother, he did share that he would not expect her to live more than six months. And so, the countdown began.

In my mom's distress, she would say, "You don't know what the doctor said. I can't talk about it because I don't want to upset anyone." In other words, 'You don't know the burden I'm carrying, and I am carrying it all alone.'

I sat face to face, eye to eye with her, held her hands, and told her she would not upset me. I told her I wanted to talk about it. I let her share what she believed, and I shared that I had spoken to the doctor and that he said she was frail but did not say she had only weeks to live. Her relief was immediate (for now).

Taking a more practical approach, Dad asked, "Why is she afraid? She knows God's grace is real; she has nothing to fear."

Although that is true, there is still a fear of the unknown—the fear of a new season, a fear of a journey you will take alone.

"I imagine that when we are face-to-face with 'the end', the doubts grow louder, questioning our salvation, faith, and beliefs."

Mom and I had several conversations about the promises of God.

Admittedly, this is hard to talk about. Your prayer today may be, 'Help us to know you understand our fear and help us to turn to you when we cannot voice those fears.'

Today is a good day to thank God that He is everlasting, and His promises are true. He sees our doubts and fears and stands in the gap. He knows our faults, weaknesses, and lack of faith, and still promises life-eternal.

But when I am afraid, I will put my confidence in you. Yes, I will trust the promises of God. And since I am trusting him, what can mere man do to me?
~Psalms 56:3-4 TLB

God's Promises

For it is by grace you have been saved, through faith—and this is not from yourselves, it is the gift of God—not by works, so that no one can boast.
~ Ephesians 2:8-9 NIV

What a God he is! How perfect in every way! All his promises prove true. He is a shield for everyone who hides behind him. ~ Psalms 18:30 TLB

God has given us eternal life, and this life is in his Son. Whoever has the Son has life;
~ 1 John 5:11b-12a NIV

My sheep listen to my voice; I know them, and they follow me. I give them eternal life, and they shall never perish; no one will snatch them out of my hand.
~ John 10:27-28 NIV

If we confess our sins, he is faithful and just and will forgive us our sins and purify us from all unrighteousness. ~ 1 John 1:9 NIV

See what great love the Father has lavished on us, that we should be called children of God! And that is what we are! The reason the world does not know us is that it did not know him. Dear friends, now we are children of God, and what we will be has not yet been made known. But we know that when Christ appears, we shall be like him, for we shall see him as he is. All who have this hope in him purify themselves, just as he is pure. ~ 1 John 3:1-3 NIV

Standing in the Gap

"Standing in the gap" is a powerful practice my husband (Kelly) and I discovered by accident. It involves using God to bridge the gap between us when our words, emotions, egos, or heartache create a divide.

During tumultuous times, vocalizing our prayers to God for each other, our relationship, forgiveness, and shortcomings helped us to mend the divide.

Once we've vocalized our shortcomings with each other and God through prayer, holding onto anger, selfishness, egotism, or unforgiveness is not easy.

Two can stand back-to-back and conquer; three is even better, for a triple-braided cord is not easily broken. ~Ecclesiastes 4:12b NLT

There were moments when my mom's mind lacked clarity, and her fear and frustration got the best of her, causing hurtful repercussions for my father. Despite knowing that she wasn't herself, her words still stung and often broke his heart.

After one such incident, they were not speaking to each other, I urged my dad to join Bible devotions. (Side note: My dad is an avid Bible reader and would never say 'no' to devotions. -I admit, it was a bit of a trick.)

Although both were reluctant participants, I prayed that we would give each other grace and bridge the gap caused by biting words and heightened emotions.

Following me, Dad reluctantly agreed to pray. He reached for Mom's hand, and I left the room.

Soon enough, they were talking again about my dad's most recent project in his shop, this was their love language.

"If my people, who are called by my name, will humble themselves and pray and seek my face and turn from their wicked ways, then I will hear from heaven, and I will forgive their sin and will heal their land"
~2 Chronicles 7:14

At some point, Mom requested Dad read her the Bible and pray with her daily. And what started as a once-a-day practice turned into twice-a-day. Mom missed Dad a lot, with so many of us at the house, Dad could easily slip away to his projects, and Mom often accused him of not wanting to be with her. I wonder now if Mom's request had a dual purpose, the second was to spend more undivided time with Dad – knowing his devotion and love for reading the Bible.

I often turned to prayer, which helped me navigate difficult conversations with Mom.

Today, consider addressing the 'elephant' in the room. What have you been avoiding? What is causing emotional stress or getting in the way? How can you invite God to stand in the gap? How can you openly ask God to give you grace for the hurts and frustrations of caregiving?

The Weary Caregiver

My 88-year-old father was my mom's primary caregiver, and although he was weary, his service to her was a labor of love.

Caregiving is not for the 'faint of heart;' stress and exhaustion can be life-threatening it is important to identify your support system early.

I have four siblings, and we quickly recognized the need to relieve Dad as often as possible. A trip to the grocery store or an opportunity to mow the lawn was a welcome reprieve.

We held family meetings to discuss our parents' needs and identify who could do what. It's important to understand that all talents are not created equal. While one sibling might handle most of the caregiving, another might be better suited for running errands and making meals.

My sister Jeannine has extensive caregiving experience and became essential in Mom's day-to-day care. She worked from our parents' home 3–4 days a week and gave my dad much-needed overnight support.

At the same time, my sister Laura spent more time with Mom than with her husband for nine straight months. She was a constant companion to Mom and did everything she could to support Mom and Dad.

My sister Doreen never heard a need she didn't try to fulfill. She purchased things that made the journey easier and cooked enough to feed an army regularly.

My brother Bill could not offer direct caregiving but was consistently at our parent's home to help Dad with household needs.

We were all there at various times; some spent the night, and others for dinner and cards. Incidentally, I had my fill of seeing my family in their skivvies.

One evening, Jeannine and I were spending the night when we overheard Mom having trouble. We both jumped out of bed and hurried to our parents' room. Together, we reasoned with Mom and worked through her crisis. Once the crisis passed, Dad glanced over, only to be met with my 60-year-old sister Jeannine dressed head-to-toe in bright yellow SpongeBob pajamas. With his trademark dry, monotone delivery, Dad deadpanned, "Nice pajamas." Once again, laughter ensued.

Do not fear, for I have redeemed you; I have summoned you by name; you are mine. When you pass through the waters, I will be with you;

and when you pass through the rivers, they will not sweep over you. When you walk through the fire, you will not be burned; the flames will not set you ablaze.
~Isaiah 43:1b - 2 NIV

It is not uncommon for families to become angry or even estranged while caring for a loved one. When one person feels like another is not doing their part, it is infuriating - especially amidst the weariness.

There are a few things to consider:

- We are not all equipped with the same talents and abilities.

- Some are better and more confident at seeing what needs to be done and taking action.

- It is rare for someone to understand the depth of caregiving unless they are doing it, and words cannot sufficiently explain it, it's better not to try.

Here are some things you might do:

- Work to give each other grace, every moment, every day.

- Pray together; it's difficult to remain angry at someone you are praying with or for.

- Discuss needs and abilities regularly as a family—do it before the situation becomes dire, as needs can change swiftly.

- Understand that there is more than one way to do things (this is hard for me).

- Pick your battles.

- If a sibling cannot help physically, they might contribute financially to pay for extra help.

- Take advantage of all services available through the healthcare system.

- When someone offers to help, be specific with your instructions. Remember, what seems like an obvious next step to you may not be clear to others.

It's difficult to remain open-minded, kind, and gracious when tired and angry.

The caregiving journey has multiple layers and many unexpected twists and turns that require flexibility and creativity.

Today, look for small ways that others can help you. Pray that God will send those people your way. Remember that not everyone will be capable of doing what you do. Explore their gifts and identify opportunities to enjoy small moments of relief. For example, consider a "patient sitter" who can stay with your loved one while you rest or complete other tasks.

He gives power to the weak
and strength to the powerless. ~Isaiah 40:29 NLT

Validate And Redirect

Mom's health took a swift turn after a heart issue required a procedure with anesthesia. She was in the hospital for several days, and when she returned home, her memory had shifted.

She often said, "I just want to go home." I responded, "Home with Jesus?" She would reply, "No, home, home."

She wanted to go back to the house my parents lived in fifteen years ago. She had no memory of moving to this new house she had lived in for the past 15 years.

She believed my father had sold the house they built and loved without her consent. She was also upset by the number of people intruding into their lives, her daughters, caregivers, nurses, and physical and occupational therapists.

I could see her point of view. She didn't remember going to the hospital. The last thing she remembered was living happily in their old home. She woke up in a place she did not recognize, surrounded by her children and strangers she did not care to entertain.

This caused her great distress and added extra heartache for my father. On one occasion, she tearfully and painfully looked into my father's eyes and said, "I'm not mad, but I am so hurt that you didn't even talk to me about it."

The hurt and confusion in my father's eyes were something I had never seen. He tried to reason with her to no avail. She explained that she loved having the girls (her daughters) around but was hurt because no one discussed it with her.

She was talking about selling the house, which didn't happen. I stepped in to redirect, addressing the number of people coming and going, and I took the blame. I was the one who insisted on every bit of healthcare service we could get, bringing a continual stream of healthcare workers into her life daily.

By accepting the blame, validating her feelings, and not trying to convince her she was wrong, her unease, concern, and anger began to fade.

She asked what had happened to her. We explained that she had been in the hospital and underwent a procedure that affected her memory. She accepted this explanation at that moment, and although this was not the end of the accusations, it was the beginning of her resolve. Eventually, accepting the loss of memory and often asking how she got here. At one point, she even asked what she had missed, and we had fun revisiting the events of the past 15 years.

After hearing the stories multiple times, she began to believe them, and this part of our troubling journey subsided while new concerns arose.

My sister Laura still hurts because Mom called her a liar. Mom insisted Laura was trying to kill her by giving her more pills than prescribed. It was not the first time we had to call on reinforcements at midnight to convince her she was not in danger.

Sharing these stories, I am deeply moved by Mom's vulnerability. She was an assertive, spirited woman, and while a large part of that strength remained, I found myself deeply drawn to the new, sweet, soft, sensitive side of her.

My mother's memory loss was vastly different from severe dementia or Alzheimer's. These two diseases add additional burden to the caregiver or family.

Learn to accept your loved one's current truth. Lengthy explanations or corrections will not serve you or your loved one. Learn to redirect or, when appropriate, step into the fantasy and enjoy the moment.

Look for new ways to keep your loved one occupied. My mother could no longer hold the storyline in movies she used to love. Instead, they agitated her because she would doze off and wake up unable to follow the story. I learned that the cooking shows (especially the children) and ice skating held her attention longer, and if she dozed off, it was easy to reconnect. She also loved gardening and birds, which made picture-filled books and magazines a perfect pastime. Watching Mom flip through a magazine often brought me back to simpler times—it felt so wonderfully 'normal.'

Do not underestimate the power of music. I used a Google Mini to turn on music at any time. Music is not only calming, it is nostalgic. My mom asked for the music regularly.

One evening, at 3 AM, I came across a random Pandora station that Mom enjoyed. She rested easily in a chair, listening to the music. The next day, she insisted I find the same "station" - impossible with a random Pandora station. And so it goes; one small victory brings on a new challenge.

Doreen bought Mom a CD player and a CD she loved. She began listening to the same CD every night on repeat while she fell asleep. This was a workable solution for soothing her to sleep. However, without a hearing aid, it played at max volume, and my sisters also listened to the same CD night after night at max volume via the baby monitor. It was like being stuck in the mall at Christmas, endlessly listening to Mariah Carey's "All I Want for

Christmas Is You." One small victory brings on a new challenge.

What worked today may or may not work tomorrow, but it might work again a week from now. The secret is to keep trying and stay creative and innovative.

There is a good chance someone else has faced a comparable situation. No caregiver is an island—find resources to support you mentally and physically.

Pray today for wisdom and guidance as you navigate the daily tug of uncertainty. And if all you have are tears and exhaustion, He knows your heart and needs.

My tears are the words with which I tell God,
my pain
Adolfo Quesada.

Creating Solutions

Full-time caregiving is a heavy lift, a constant challenge to stay one step ahead of the unforeseen dangers lurking just around the corner.

One evening, my dad woke up to find my mom in the bathroom, cleaning out under the sink. She wasn't sure how she got there and couldn't remember it by morning. This incident made her overly concerned that she had been sleepwalking and might hurt herself at night. It led to a new dilemma: trying to catch her as she moved from the bed at night.

The simplest solution would have been a guard rail, but in our situation, Mom was too weak to crawl into bed herself which required us to use a thin mattress cover to slide her across the bed into place from the opposite side. Even a drop bed rail was impractical—it got in the way and could not be safely positioned once she was in bed.

I also explored the idea of using an infrared beam along the base of the floor that would sound an alarm if her foot crossed it. I had seen this solution work successfully for another family, but unfortunately, I couldn't find a similar setup that worked for us.

We tried many ideas with little success until I had the most brilliant idea of buying a motion detector alarm, which you might use for intruders.

My dad and I worked together to set it up exactly right. Dad held it on the bedside table, adjusting the detector ever so slightly repeatedly as I rolled back and forth and back and forth and back and forth across the bed to achieve the perfect angle that would capture my mom as she reached the edge of the bed. After 60 to 90 minutes, we were satisfied and proud of ourselves.

Have I mentioned that my father is very deaf without his hearing aids? Although he slept with one hearing aid, he set the alarm to a loud firehouse alarm to ensure he would hear it.

That evening, I woke to a slight noise in my parents' room, as I quietly and slowly slid the door open to peek into the room, a five-alarm firehouse siren went off at sonic boom levels. My mom and dad shot out of bed like rockets.

In the next 10 seconds, utter chaos ensued. I couldn't turn it off since it was an intruder alarm, and I was the intruder. My dad fumbled for the remote, and finally, there was silence, other than the pounding of our hearts and, eventually, uncontrollable laughter.

I still laugh aloud as I share this story. It will remain a family favorite, forever embedded in my mind. The scene was epic.

We had failed to evaluate the detector's full 110-degree range, which included the door. The alarm was promptly returned to Amazon. Not so brilliant.

Our final solution was to move a wing chair next to the bed once Mom was settled in bed.

Let us not become weary in doing good, for at the proper time we will reap a harvest if we do not give up. ~ Galatians 6:9

As I mentioned, my mom had lost quite a bit of weight, so much that it hurt her to sit or lie down because she was all bone. Our daily and nightly challenge became finding ways to keep her comfortable. During the day, we frequently adjusted her chair, cushions, and position, trying to find just the right combination. At night, after midnight, when she was ready for bed, it could take hours to help her settle. She often said there were rocks in her bed.

We tried body pillows, wedge pillows, memory foam mattresses, cozy blankets, and more with marginal success. What worked one night might not work the next. Some nights, we couldn't find any solution. Just as Dad would settle into bed, Mom would need to go to the bathroom, and the entire process would start over again. After two or three hours, when Dad was exhausted and frustrated, I (or one of my sisters) would take Mom to the living room, where we'd sit up the rest of the night listening to music and dozing together.

I searched social media sites for anorexia support groups hoping someone there might have discovered a wonderful solution but nothing.

We also tried sleep aids, relaxation medication, antidepressants, and eventually pain medication to help her (and my dad) find relief and get rest.

Unfortunately, there is no 'one-size-fits-all' solution in caregiving, it is a daily struggle of trial and error.

If you have been caring for a loved one, you know that laughter is essential. Late at night, my sisters and I often found ourselves giggling at the disjointed exchanges between our two hard-of-hearing parents, captured through the baby monitor—it went something like this:

> Mom (sweetly): "Do you have enough blankets?"
> Dad (kindly): "You need another blanket; I'll get one." (leaves the room to fetch a blanket)
> Mom (angrily): "Why did you walk out on me?"

Dad (perplexed by her sudden anger, cautiously drapes another blanket over her)

Mom (still upset): "That's too many blankets!"

Dad (puzzled, removes the extra blanket and climbs back into bed)

Mom (sweetly): "Thank you, I love you."

Dad (a little grumpy): "What?"

Mom (louder and with less sweetness): "I said, thank you, I love you."

Dad (bothered): "What?"

Mom (resigned): "Never mind"

What started as a sweet interaction ended in frustration.

Come to me, all who labor and are heavy laden, and I will give you rest. ~Matthew 11:28 NIV

Where are you heavy laden? Maybe it's in the rush, not slowing down enough to hear the sweet words of your loved one. Perhaps it's the expectation of harsh words, or maybe you've built a wall around your heart that protects but also dulls your hearing. Patience is difficult especially when we are tired, hungry, overworked, and dismayed.

Years ago, I cared for a lovely woman who was rarely harsh but could be stubborn and difficult. Yet on rare occasions, as I put her to bed, she would look up at me and say, "I love you." In those moments, every hard part of the day would dissolve with those three simple words.

Today is a good day to slow down, breathe, and actively listen for sweet words. Ask God to help you recognize those short, tender moments that often hide within the walls of chaos. And when your loved one is quiet and calm, embrace the silence and know they are saying, "Thank you, I love you."

Cherished Memories

When I shared with others that Mom was sick, the doctor expected her to live no longer than six months, and the family joined together to care for her, I suspect that people imagined her lying in bed, gravely ill, and near death. This could not be further from the truth.

Mom was up daily, cleaned up, dressed, and in a chair.

Every evening, the family would gather to play cards. Mom was limited to the games she could play, but the games all started the same way.

Mom: (confused) "I've never played this game."

Family: (helping her) "Play this, play that."

Mom: (agitated) "You have to remember; I'm just learning this game."

Family: (helping her) "Play this, play that."

Mom (irritably and matter of fact): "You act like I've never played this game before; I have a brain in my head."

.... Mom wins again!

Mom often felt like she couldn't do anything. We worked to find ways to keep her engaged. Sometimes it worked beautifully, and sometimes, not so much.

With our six months ticking away, we decided on two projects to make the most of these days:

1. Create a memory book to honor Mom and Dad and the life they built.
2. Create a family Christmas to remember.

Luckily, my mom had their 65 years of photos well organized, some on 35-mm slides. We spent night after night sitting together watching family slide shows, laughing, sharing, and trying to figure out 'who the heck is that kid?" We took note of special memories and selected photos worthy of entering the memory book.

This occupied many evenings and was a beautiful way to spend time as a family. A few months later, Mom and Dad's 65th wedding anniversary, the 50-page memory book arrived in print.

What's equally important regarding the memory book is that it was a tool to use every day. Whether we were sitting with Mom, or she was sitting alone, it was a beautiful way to occupy time, share memories, and bring a happy, positive spin to the day.

Bonus: it has also served my father beautifully as he mourns the loss of his wife and life as he knew it.

Today, pull out some photos to share. You do not need a memory book. If your photos are on your phone, cast them on the TV; the most significant part of this activity is the time, and memories shared and if your loved one has memory loss, this activity can happen day after day.

A Christmas to Remember

Like so many people, Mom loved Christmas, a time to gather, share love through gift-giving, play games, laugh, and build memories. One moment in time when the whole family slowed long enough to eat, play, and laugh together. Each year, the family grew, and this dream became increasingly more difficult to attain - do you know teenagers and young people?

This year, the last year we would celebrate Christmas with Mom, our goal was to give her that dream, those precious moments when the world slowed down; a time when we all showed up, sat in the same room, and enjoyed the moment for what it was.

We planned for weeks, and although Mom didn't always remember the plan, she was right in the middle of the action, sharing ideas and planning three matching events on three different days. This allowed everyone to visit while keeping the groups more intimate, and less taxing. We set up games in the living room, right in front of Mom's chair, allowing her to play along. We hung Mom's old Christmas ornaments on a bare tree branch that served as Christmas gifts to all who attended. As each family member left, they chose an ornament gift from Mom.

Although the day was technically for Mom, as I look at it now, I realize it was really for each of us. As each event wrapped up and grandchildren said their goodbyes, most knew this was the final goodbye.

On New Year's Eve, Mom was in rare form; midnight was her favorite hour these days. We played games, told stories, sang, wore red noses, and laughed. My heart is still brimming; it was an incredible night. This is a magical memory I will never forget, and it would not have happened if I had been more worried about the dishes in the sink, sorting weekly meds, or the clothes in the washer.

While wearing our red noses, we sang *You Are My Sunshine* to each other. Although I cannot believe I will ever forget it, I am pleased it was recorded.

We are so blessed to have so many memorable moments.

Memories are made in the small moments of everyday life.

What is disheartening about being a caregiver is that you no longer get to be spouse, child, grandchild, etc.

You are consumed with caring and too tired to be much of anything else.

This is why Bible devotions, reflection, and gratitude in the morning are so powerful. Time alone with your loved one to chat and connect, if only for a few minutes.

Of course, having support makes disconnecting easier. If you have no family support, try stepping away when the healthcare worker is visiting. I know this is hard when you are the 24/7 keeper of all things, you start to think and talk for your loved one and believe they are not safe without you in the room; I can relate.

However, what will your loved one do if you suffer a medical issue due to stress, lack of sleep, and exhaustion?

I also understand the inevitable dilemma; you plan to get up earlier to grab a shower and, hello, monkey wrench.

Think mini vacations, mini moments of relaxation, mini moments of deep breathing, mini moments of fresh air, mini moments of laughter. Self-care is critical and does not have to be a day at the spa or someone coming to relieve you for an entire week (although that would be a great gig if you could get it).

The tasks and the toilet can wait. Figure out how to step back, let go of the caregiver's hat, play a game, look at photos, laugh, share stories, whatever allows you to connect as a loved one rather than the keeper of the rules.

How can you make today a special day? Memories are made in the small moments of everyday life. I hope you will find time today to step away from being the caregiver and be the loved one.

Pray for God to reveal moments of opportunity to relax, reflect, laugh, and just be. You might enjoy some sunshine or get your hands in the garden rather than in the dishes—or spend time knitting, sewing, reading, or doing whatever helps you breathe a little easier.

The Gray Area

Living in the gray or fuzzy comes effortlessly to some but not necessarily to others. It means to let go of the black and white, let go of the right and wrong, explore and enjoy the moment, and let it develop into whatever it is.

If your loved one has memory loss, you know what the gray area looks like. It is like the moments between sleep, dreams, and reality—when the dream makes sense.

Although it takes only seconds for us to realize that this was a dream and it has no basis, loved ones with memory loss may live in this space for extended periods.

You have two choices, spend your day trying to correct them and agitate yourself and them, or go with the flow and let the conversation go where it goes regardless of its reality.

It reminds me of one of my favorite movies, "House Sitters." with Goldie Hawn and Steve Martin. The movie is built on fantasies created at the moment by Goldie Hawn, while Steve Martin tries to bring everything back to truth and reality; joy and love are discovered when he steps into the fantasy with her.

If you have not seen it, watch it, and then go ahead and live in the fantasy.

One of my first experiences with 'the gray area' was with a gentle elderly man who often told me he had received a call from the president that morning and we would be flying out that afternoon on Air Force One to meet with him.

I loved delving into the conversation and asking what he thought the president might need from him. The answers were different each time, but the conversation was still fun. It made his wife crazy that he said it and that I entertained it. But what did it hurt? It's not like I was driving him to the airport. Later in the day, if he persisted, I might tell him the president called to reschedule.

Another fun experience was with my wonderful friend Connie. During our daily car rides in Spring, she would comment, "Oh, look at how green the trees are." On the third or fourth day of this routine, before she had a chance, I would say, "Oh. look at how green the trees are." She would respond, "I was just thinking that".

I also love the gray area for what I can read between the lines.

On one occasion, my mom was folding and unfolding a blanket on her lap and started to refer to it as medication. Although this didn't make sense, we were in the gray area. The conversation turned to tracking medications, and she asked each of us if we had taken our daily medications.

The conversation went something like this:

Mom: (questioning) "Did you take your medication today?"

Family: (all answering at once)

Mom: (matter of fact and pointing a finger at us) "Answer one at a time."

Me: (definitively) "I don't take medication."

Mom: (stern voice) "That's not what I asked. I asked if you took your medication."

Mom: (strictly) "Now did you take your medication."

Bill: (assuredly) "I took vitamins."

Mom: (sternly): "That's not what I asked. I asked if you took your medication."

Laura: (timidly) "I took one of my medications but not the other."

Mom: (still stern): "I did not ask what you didn't take. I asked what you did take."

This continued around and around in the same manner, and we egged it on. Mom then began to tell me I needed to track medications every day.

> Me: (questioning) "I need to track everyone's medication?"

> Mom: (directly) "Yes, get paper and pen."

I got paper and pen, and Mom started giving me instructions on how to track medications.

> Me: (challenging) "Why should I have to track their meds?"

> Mom: (authoritatively) "Just do it!"

At some point, my father walked in, and with confusion, he told my mother it was a blanket, not medication. We gave Dad a look to play along, and he also shared that he had taken his meds.

This was so humorous, and three days after the incident, Dad and my siblings continued to report to me that they had taken their meds.

Interestingly, the palliative nurse explained that patients often try to process things in their minds as they prepare to leave.

I don't know if that's what Mom was doing if she was trying to teach us something, or if it was just a gray moment.

I do know that no humans or animals were hurt, my mom got to express herself, and our family shared additional bonding moments.

Today is a good day to ask God to allow your defenses to relax and your sense of humor to take the lead. Ask Him to remind you to let the moments unfold naturally and to appreciate the exact place you are with your loved one.

Work to abandon the black and white and live in the gray when it doesn't matter - Don't sweat the small stuff, and it's all small stuff.

Dance and swing let your heart sing.

For everything there is a season, a time for every activity under heaven. A time to be born and a time to die. A time to plant and a time to harvest...A time to cry and a time to laugh. A time to grieve and a time to dance...Yet God has made everything beautiful for its own time.
~ Ecclesiastes 3 NLT

Words of Joy

In the last 24 hours of Mom's life, she was primarily nonverbal. My sister Laura sat by her bed, held her hand, and silently pleaded, "I just want to hear her say 'I love you' once more."

In those same final days, my brother Bill sat with Mom. She grasped his hands and looked into his eyes intently. I'm not sure my brother caught what she was saying with her eyes, but I heard it loud and clear. There was so much love in her gaze, and I know she was urging him and each of us: "Live life to the fullest, find happiness, don't let your sorrows define you, get back up, go do what you were made to do, and I'm proud of you."

I called Mom daily during those last months. We always said "I love you" as we said goodbye. Occasionally, she would say, "I love you, Dianne," and my heart soared. I loved hearing her say my name. I only wish I had a recording of it. Hearing someone say your name in love is like hearing your name lifted in prayer—it is grand.

Words are significant; they have power, and they matter. They hold the dynamic ability to light up a life or break a heart.

Some people express themselves and their feelings better than others. Today is the day to let God 'stand in the gap.' Step outside your comfort zone, say what's in your heart, and express your feelings.

Find your words, express yourself fully, and share words of joy in your prayer with God and your loved one:

- God, thank you for [name]. Thank you for the love that we share, the time we have experienced, the lessons we have learned.

- I know I don't say it enough; thank you for helping us find each other.

- I am thankful that we get to share this life.

- I am not particularly good at sharing my feelings; help me to share my thoughts and feelings.

- I am sorry for the sorrow I have caused; help me to be what [name] needs today.

- Please help me to forgive and to ask for forgiveness.

- I love you, God, and I love [name].

- Please help us to forgive each other easily and to give each other grace today.

Just like cream rises to the top, your sweetest and finest memories will also rise to the top. Old hurts will be forgotten, and you will be left with cherished souvenirs of a love gone by.

Two days after my mother passed, I was sitting with my father who shared, "As frustrated as I was at times, I miss her so much."

The time is now! Do not underestimate the profound impact of your words; speak boldly and confidently with words of love, gratitude, and compassion.

Transitions

My niece Jennifer, Laura's daughter, the first grandchild, and Mom's you-are-my-world relationship discovered a set of five small booklets that explained what to expect at each stage of end-of-life care. * It would not be uncommon to find one or more of us curled up in the living room, absorbed in these books. I am not sure why this surprised me, but it did. We each cared deeply about what to expect and how we might serve and support Mom better. This information helped us to move seamlessly together. The pure love expressed through this act was not lost on me.

When the doctor suggested we consult palliative care, the same was true. Five of us piled into the small exam room to listen, understand, and participate in the palliative care conversation, recording it to share with those not there.

Palliative care is not hospice. It is a continuum of care for patients with serious illnesses that have moved from a goal of cure to a maintenance goal. Palliative care helps manage numerous aspects of medication, doctors, and more.

We did not know what to expect, but I loved how the palliative nurse spoke directly to Mom. She asked how she was feeling and what her desires were.

Mom wasn't exactly sure how to respond. Until then, we rarely asked Mom what she wanted except what she wanted to eat. She was losing weight weekly, and our goal was to have her consume 1,000 calories daily to maintain her weight. Additionally, we managed and distributed medication, encouraged exercise, and took on her care as our full-time job.

Eventually, Mom responded that she wanted everyone to stop bossing her around. She said it in jest, and we all laughed—we did boss her around, but that's what had to be done to keep her alive.

By the end of the conversation, we realized how much truth was in Mom's jest.

The nurse shared that it was time to let Mom's body do what it needed to do. She explained that her body knew what to do and probably would not need 1,000 calories daily. Mom would know when enough was enough.

From then on, she got to decide what to eat or drink; we had to remind each other regularly that she got to decide.

It's hard when you believe your loved one's actions will lead to the end. But what is better than allowing them to die as they lived—on their terms?

When Mom would often complain of pain or a distressing day, my answer was always the same; "Mom, you get to decide. When there are more bad days than good days, that's when you say, 'enough'."

Day after day, Mom chose life. She often acknowledged she was being selfish or complaining and apologized for it.

Today's prayer may be one of the hardest. Ask God for guidance and wisdom to let go of control. Ask for ears that hear your loved one's requests and continue to keep the lines of communication open, asking them regularly what they want.

Walking In Their Shoes

The closer she got to heaven's gates, the more she needed my father nearby, constantly. Although my dad enjoys a nap in front of the TV, he is often on the go with several projects in the works. Did I tell you about the beautiful cedar chest he stripped and refinished for her for their 65th wedding anniversary? -gorgeous.

He could barely leave the room without her calling out. He took up reading mystery novels and managed to read through my mother's book-of-the-month library while he sat with her.

In the evening, they would sit side-by-side on the couch, holding hands, watching TV, and dozing until the stroke of midnight, and Mom was willing to go to bed.

Patience, understanding, and gentleness can be challenging when your heart hurts and your good intentions are met with anger or abuse.

Luckily for our family, Mom often knew when she had been abusive, and at some point, after the moment had passed, she would apologize. This is not always true for all loved ones, and the abuse keeps on coming without relief and can quickly wear the caregiver's heart and soul down.

Jeannine drove two hours to support Dad and be with Mom, typically staying for 3-4 days at a time. On one occasion in the middle of her stay, Mom said, "Don't you have a home to go to? Why don't you go home?" On another occasion, Mom said, "Do you mind if I spend some time alone with my husband?"

As I've shared earlier, there was no such thing as alone time in our family.

In both instances, Jeannine was wise enough not to react and went to her room, leaving Mom alone. But it doesn't mean it didn't hurt.

When words pierce your heart, it hurts, and somehow you must figure out how to regroup and move on in love.

Today, you might ask God to help you be gentle and loving in the face of your loved one's vulnerability. Ask God for a deeper level of patience, understanding, and forgiveness as the needs and demands of your loved one become greater.

Adding meditation (not medication) and journaling to your self-care may be surprisingly rewarding.

I am worn out from my groaning. All night long I flood my bed with weeping and drench my couch with tears. ~ *Psalms 6:6 NIV*

I'll Think About That Tomorrow

As my 60-day stay came to an end, Mom's condition changed only slightly each day. She continued to lose weight, and sometimes she would sleep well into the afternoon—so much so that I would creep in to check on her, fearful she might have stopped breathing.

One afternoon, while Mom sat dozing, she suddenly shot up urgently and told me to give her the walker. I asked her what she needed, and she said, "They just called me. Didn't you hear them?"

My first thought wasn't the 'gray area,' but that someone was calling her home!

After three seconds of panic, I calmly said to the room, "Whoever is here with her right now, thank you for being here. Help her to stay calm, and please take care of her."

"The angel of the Lord encamps around those who fear him, and delivers them"
~Psalms 34:7 NIV

"For he will order his angels to protect you wherever you go, and they will hold you up with their hands, so

you won't even hurt your foot on a stone".
~Psalms 91:11-12 NLT

I know it sounds crazy, but in those brief moments, it felt right. I imagined one of Mom's sisters, my brother, or her good friend Maureen might be with her.

Before I left, I wanted to make sure as many details as possible were handled. I researched and chose a funeral home, made sure the DNR (Do Not Resuscitate) was in order and available, and wrote the obituary.

I was able to remain somewhat removed as I researched and chose the funeral home, but when faced with paperwork that required me to add Mom's name in the deceased field. I couldn't do it. That just made it too real. I left that to be completed when the time came.

One precious gem of information I learned from the funeral home was that we did not have to call anyone for up to eight hours once Mom passed. We tucked this information in the back of our minds, and it was invaluable later.

It was impossible to stay detached as I created the obituary. I had written many obituaries and funeral services in the past, but never for someone so close to my heart. It was heart-wrenching. I completed it and stored it with the funeral paperwork and DNR before I left.

A few years before Mom passed, we, the family, sat around the table and discussed Mom and Dad's wishes. It wasn't an easy conversation, but I can't imagine what it would have been like if we had waited until we got the six-month notice.

Today might be a good day to have those conversations. If they are grueling, try just a few questions a day. Also, make use of devotion time for this.

Gentle Activities and Questions to Start a Last Wishes Conversation:

- Play Hymns: During devotions, play hymns via phone, CD, or Google Mini. Sing along and share your favorite hymn. Ask your loved one about their favorite hymn. If they don't know, remind them of some old-time favorites. Google search favorite hymns or best funeral hymns to get some ideas.

- Favorite Bible Verses: Google 'favorite Bible verses', read the verses as part of devotions, and ask which ones are their favorites.

- Family History: Start a conversation about their family history—parents, siblings, aunts, uncles, children, etc. Ask them to share their favorite memories. Use pictures to stir the discussion. This can lead to a wonderful conversation.

- Discussing Burial Preferences: As you discuss family history, consider asking about the dates of passing, cremation details, and burial locations of family members. Share your preferences as well; this can help ease into a conversation about your loved one's wishes regarding cremation and burial.

- Lighthearted Jokes: My husband and I joke about scattering his ashes at Yankee Memorial Park—this is his dream, not to be buried next to me, but to be forever with Babe Ruth. You can use this same lighthearted approach to joke about where you or they might want to be scattered, such as at a BINGO hall, a college football field, Hawaii, or an ex-husband's front yard.

Remember to be curious, not interrogative. Enjoy this time, laugh together, and take notes.

There is Truth in The Gray Area

During the last devotion time with Mom, before I left, we thanked God for the time we had spent together, and Mom prayed, "Thank you for Dianne; she has been so sweet." - words of joy.

I went to bed early that night but could not sleep. I was leaving at 4 AM, and I knew my goodnight hug and cuddles with Mom could be my last goodbye. I lay in bed, crying most of the night, willing myself to sleep to no avail.

At 3 AM, I wandered out of the bedroom to find Mom and Laura awake in the living room. Mom wouldn't go to bed, and Laura was held captive, unable to leave Mom alone.

I cuddled with Mom for another 30 minutes before tearing myself away. As I stepped outside to pack my car, I found Dad clearing it and plowing the driveway. A snowstorm that was supposed to clear the day before continued. I had already waited out the storm for two days. I got in my car and slowly and sadly pulled out of the driveway.

My heart broke as I drove away, knowing I shouldn't be behind the wheel. It was dark, snowing, and slippery, and I was exhausted and crying—a dangerous combination. To make matters worse, the washer fluid in my Florida car wasn't suitable for New York's cold, leaving my windshield a salty, grimy mess and impairing my vision. If ever God needed to take the wheel, it was this day.

Once home, I returned to work, though my heart remained in New York as my siblings took turns caring for Mom and supporting Dad. I talked to Mom most days, and when she said, "No, I don't want to talk to anyone," I bullied my way in and told her she had no choice.

During one phone call, Mom was spitting and sputtering because Dad had used a big dollop of adhesive on her dentures. She was in the bathroom trying to get it out of her mouth and off her teeth. I was laughing, but she was not.

While in the gray area, Mom had mentioned a dentist more than once. I didn't think much of this until late in her care when keeping her teeth in her mouth became impossible. As it turns out, weight loss had caused her gum line to shrink, and her teeth didn't fit. - who knew?

She had complained about being unable to chew some of her favorite foods, and we never made a connection. Our first clue should have been when she stopped eating maple walnut ice cream because there were too many walnuts. Is that even possible? Too many walnuts?

We finally called a dentist and discovered they could readjust dentures to fit. She had an appointment she never made; she got a new set of teeth in heaven.

Today, ask God to help you hear the truths within the gray area. To give you wisdom to see what your loved one needs. You might pray together that you would recognize the unspoken needs between you. Mom often noticed how weary Dad looked and would encourage him to rest. It might surprise you to hear the prayers of your loved one for your needs.

The Rally

The palliative care nurse, Robert, started his visits shortly after I left. Although he initially wasn't sure his services were necessary, his weekly visits provided peace of mind, especially for Dad.

Mom knew the decision to go into hospice was hers. One evening on the phone, she asked, "Do you think choosing hospice is like committing suicide?"

My heart hurt because of her internal struggle. I reassured her, explaining that she would stop taking daily medications and only take medications to make her comfortable. But God was still in control.

This satisfied her, and she continued to choose life for several weeks.

A few weeks before Mom passed, we were talking on the phone, and she told me she was ready. I told her that was okay, and we would discuss it with Robert on Thursday.

On Thursday, I was on speakerphone while Mom, Dad, my siblings, and Robert gathered around the same table where we had celebrated holidays and dinners for years.

I was attending a conference when the call came in, so I stepped into the courtyard to answer it. I listened as my father updated Robert on the week's events and discussed Mom's ongoing care. Finally, I interrupted, saying, 'Robert, the reason we're all here is that Mom has decided to move into hospice.'

Robert immediately began to explain the steps that would take place. Moving did not mean relocating Mom; it just meant transferring her file from palliative care to hospice care—she would stay at home.

Before moving forward, I said, "Let's include Mom and ensure this is what she wants." I expected Robert, the trained palliative nurse, to handle this, but instead, the phone was pushed in front of Mom, and someone said, "Go ahead, Dianne. Mom has the phone."

Through tears, I said, "Mom, the reason we are all here is because you said you are ready to go into hospice. That means all your medications will stop, nurses will make you comfortable, and God will decide what's next. How does that sound?"

Quieting my cries, I listened to Mom's response. Very matter of fact, she said, "I don't think so. I want the preacher to preach on me a little bit more."

In the public courtyard, I erupted into sobs and laughter. A short reprieve! -I'll take it.

A week later, on Thursday, my sister called to tell me Mom was moving to hospice. I was on a plane and home that evening.

We learned Friday that hospice care was unable to move Mom's care until Monday; we were on our own until then.

Today is a good day to pray for wisdom and strength. No matter how difficult the road has been so far, the hardest part of the journey is just beginning.

The Last Goodbye

The next few days are a blur. We had no idea Mom would go so fast. She was gone less than 72 hours after deciding to move to hospice. I can only remember dozing for a few hours with Mom. Yet I can't remember being tired.

Friday, Mom and Dad's pastor and his wife visited. Mom sat on the side of the bed, and we encircled her physically and with great love. We prayed, sang, and shared God's promises. As this time concluded, Mom began to pray aloud in a manner I had never heard before. Over and over, she prayed, pleaded, and cried for God to forgive her for not being enough and to take her home.

As I write this, my eyes fill with tears, and my soul groans. Don't Go, please don't go!

I am worn out from sobbing. All night I flood my bed with weeping, drenching it with my tears.
~Psalms 6:6 NLT

Now, I imagine the depth of turmoil and uncertainty Mom may have suffered as her mind adjusted to what would be the end and the journey she would take—not alone, but without the hand of her lifelong partner.

Jennifer arrived on Friday, and she and I held vigil over Mom while Dad and siblings got well-deserved rest. We watched several informative YouTube videos produced by a Hospice nurse. *

Friday night, she rested for short periods. She wasn't talking much, but when Jennifer tried to adjust the pillows and accidentally knocked her on the head, she only replied, "WOW." We erupted in laughter. I love that she never lost her sense of humor.

Periodically, she would ask to stand up. We would stand her up, readjust her bed, and lay her back down.

Saturday came in like a lamb. Mom was quiet and primarily nonverbal.

Laura sat alone with her, hoping to hear her say, "I love you" one last time.

Dad sat for hours singing hymn after hymn directly from the hymnal acapella. This was a sweet and beautiful work of the heart. However, he did sound a little like a 13-year-old boy singing his Bar Mitzvah prayer.

Ironically, the lyrics to the Bar Mitzvah song tell those being celebrated to go and begin the journey they are meant to have.

We are not Jewish, but I thought that was a beautiful connection.

As Saturday night came upon us, Jennifer and I sat with Mom. She was awake most of the night but labored. She cried out often for water, and we moistened her mouth with a sterile sponge.

She would straighten up, lean forward, and violently slump back, lacking the energy to stay up. We stacked pillows behind her to help keep her upright.

We assured her that we would be okay and would take care of Dad, one of her biggest concerns.

At 12:30 AM, she leaned forward, looked beyond us, lifted her arms, and struggled to say, 'Stand up, please.' We lifted her to stand between us in a glorious three-way hug. As her body went limp, Jennifer sat back, laid her in her lap, and held her in her arms.

Dad rushed to her side and received the last squeeze of her hand.

Thanks to the information provided by the funeral home, we did not call 911 at once. Instead, we dressed her, fixed her hair, folded her arms, and added flowers to her hands.

We spent time alone with her, cuddled into her, and said our last goodbyes. We encircled her with our bodies, love, songs, and prayers.

It was an overwhelming yet awe-inspiring goodbye. Mom passed gently from our arms into Jesus' arms.

My greatest pain to date was the moment your heart stopped beating and mine continued.

Tears are all I have today, but my heart is so thankful for a God who understands me to the depths of my soul.

What Comes Next

Even today, those last moments remain vivid in my mind. As beautiful as they were, I often wish I had done things differently. For example, I wish I had recognized how close we were to the end sooner. The first call I made was to the funeral director, who instructed me to contact non-emergency 911. Here are a few lessons I learned:

- When we called non-emergency 911, paramedics arrived first. They checked her vitals and requested the DNR. The police followed, conducting their private investigation while we, the family, waited outside the closed door. Afterward, the medical examiner arrived and also required time alone with the body. What I learned is that if my mom had been officially under hospice care, there would have been no investigation. Since she wasn't, the process was necessary to rule out foul play.

- Trust your instincts. My mom was prescribed half a pain pill every 12 hours. On Friday, when I learned that hospice care wouldn't be available until Monday, I called the hospice nurse for guidance. He advised me to administer the medication every four hours, which I started immediately. By Saturday noon, I felt uneasy about the increased dosage. I called Hospice weekend support, and they insisted I revert to the original prescription. We stopped the medication, and she didn't receive any more before she passed. While I don't believe continuing the medication would have raised suspicion, I was relieved I didn't have to find out.

- After the medical examiner finished, they called the funeral director to take over.

- I had learned from a prior experience that being present when the body is transferred to the gurney is something the family might want to avoid. Watching your loved one placed on a gurney, zipped inside a body bag, can be a distressing memory. Our funeral director offered this same advice. Mom was brought out on the gurney, in a body bag that was unzipped just enough to see her face and her hands holding flowers—it was a peaceful and beautiful sight. This gave my dad the chance to share a final moment with her. Allowing him to touch, kiss, and embrace her, walking alongside her to the hearse in a tender farewell journey.

Today, I encourage you to ask God, again, for wisdom in identifying your end-of-life priorities, so that you can be intentional and present as you walk through those final moments and beyond with your loved ones.

The Aftershock

Smaller earthquakes occur in the same general area during the days to years following a larger event.

The sun rose that day as it always does, and life continued unshaken for the rest of the world. In our home, the seven of us aimlessly wandered, dazed, and changed forever.

Today was the day. I had no choice; with great heartache and agony, I wrote Mom's name in the deceased field on the funeral home paperwork.

In the days to follow, waves of sadness and tears mixed with moments of laughter hit each of us erratically,

The list of things to do seemed endless and too demanding, from final arrangements to closing credit cards to reassigning beneficiaries to eating.

As we prepared for the Celebration of Life, I felt confident in what Mom had wanted and made plans accordingly. Dad felt differently.

We went back and forth a bit, and although I conceded, I was still upset. I stomped out like a child to walk it off.

While I walked, I fussed and sputtered to God (and Mom) about being hurt and angry, wanting to honor Mom while all the time acknowledging that I was acting like a spoiled child. I rationalized my thoughts and actions, always coming back to a 'spoiled child'. Continuing my internal rant about honoring Mom, I walked by the house we grew up in—a home Mom and Dad made together, where they raised six children. And God said, "Husband trumps Daughter." (or was that my card-playing, Mom?) And "By honoring Dad, you are honoring Mom." Done. Thanks, God (and Mom).

20-second hugs to you

If you are at this point in your journey, I am so sorry for your loss and wish you 20-second hugs from the people you love and need the most right now.

Be aware of the heightened emotions of both yours and others. Each of us mourns differently; there is no right or wrong. Ask God to help you be sensitive and to offer grace to those around you. Ask Him to help you be true to yourself and to help you understand and ask for what you need.

Remember, if all you have are tears, God hears you. Words are not always necessary.

The grieving process is unique to everyone. While one person might clean out the closet immediately, another keeps everything for years. While one is stoic and manages every detail, another falls apart on the floor, unable to move forward.

There is no right or wrong; each person finds their way, and the aftershock hits differently for all.

I remained at my parent's home for two weeks, helping Dad put things in order, treasuring moments with my siblings, and holding on to the last smells and echoes of Mom's presence.

Today, I encourage you to ask God for clarity. What do you need to hold onto from your loved one? What will you cherish as you navigate the loss that will change your life forever?

The Lord is near to the brokenhearted and saves the crushed in spirit ~Psalm 34:18 NIV

Blessed are those who mourn: for they will be comforted. ~Matthew 5:4 NIV

The Disbelief of Loss

A few days after I arrived home in Florida, I sat on my couch one evening and inadvertently glanced up at a card sent by a dear friend while I was away—an 8x10 picture card of my mom. I burst into sobs.

I returned to work, not yet ready to face the world, but life requires and expects us to move on. When a colleague checked in with me, he asked how my dad was doing instead of asking how I was doing. It was brilliant; answering how I was doing would have been impossible, but asking about my dad showed me beautiful empathy and allowed me to talk about my mom without exposing the raw emotions I was still processing.

We don't always know when an aftershock will hit or why it strikes at that exact moment. It just happens. Although bursting into tears can be embarrassing and seem unprofessional, it is real, it is life, and it is a blessing to know that you loved and were loved so dearly.

As days and life moved forward, I made an uncanny discovery. My heart was undeniably shattered by the loss of this sweet, vulnerable, beautiful elderly woman whom I had grown to love even more deeply during her final six months. But in a rare moment of clarity and disbelief, I realized that I had lost my mom.

I know that sounds crazy, and I expect it goes hand in hand with the disbelief that accompanies loss, but it felt as though I lost two people. One was the vulnerable woman we cared for, and the other was my mom, the face I see in my favorite photos.

I continue to cry daily for both women and for my dad, who is trying to navigate a new norm of living without her.

Today, I pray for God to help me take this one day at a time and to hear my groans that I cannot yet put into words. I pray for our family to stay strong and continue to give each other grace as we navigate our way through grief and life without Mom. I pray that my dad finds peace and gradually discovers his new normal in the quietness of a house that is now empty.

Praise be to the Lord, to God our Savior, who daily bears our burdens. ~Psalm 68:19

We are but a Breath
A Eulogy

In the book of Psalms, David gently reminds us, 'We are but a breath,' much like the grains of sand slipping through an hourglass.

You have made my life no longer than the width of my hand. My entire lifetime is just a moment to you; at best, each of us is but a breath.
~Psalms 39:5 NLT

For they are like a breath of air; their days are like a passing shadow. ~Psalms 144:4 NLT

At an early age, Betty and her siblings found themselves in the care of the foster system. They clung to each other until they could care for each other, forging bonds of resilience and compassion for a lifetime. These formative years shaped Betty's heart; a heart of compassion and empathy, particularly for children.

As a young woman, Betty was building a bookcase in her upper apartment over an establishment Dave frequented. The owner pleaded for someone to go up and help her and stop the noise and hammering. Dave volunteered to help her, and the rest was history; he never stopped building for her.

Over the next 65 years, they became lifelong building partners. Building a life, a family, and a home (a few homes) Betty with the design ideas and Dave with the hammer and saw.

They built a family and a legacy of six children, fifteen grandchildren, and sixteen great-grandchildren. Betty devoted herself to raising her family, finding fulfillment in bridging the gaps left in her own heart.

Her home was filled with family, friends, and her sisters. The sisters often played cards from dusk till dawn, and when the kids woke up for school, they would find them still wide awake, laughing and having a wonderful time. Her doors were open to nieces, nephews, neighbors, church children, grandchildren, and more. She went above and beyond to ensure everyone enjoyed life through experiences, games, laughter, and inclusion. If you were one of those children, you were a part of her sand art.

When Betty and Dave joined Gates Community Chapel, their large family doubled the size of the congregation. But more importantly, Betty's heart expanded in size as she accepted, trusted, and began to understand the love of Jesus. Her service knew no bounds. She became affectionately known as Aunt Betty. She operated the church daycare, organized youth activities, conducted Sunday School classes, and more.

She spent over 20 years caring for troubled teens. She was Aunt Betty and a safe place for hundreds of young people, changing the landscape of their sand art forever.

Betty rarely allowed a birthday or holiday to go by without celebration. Just as the hourglass reminds us of the passage of time, she savored moments, cherished connections, and understood that life is a precious gift meant to be embraced and celebrated with joy.

As an unexpected guest at one of Betty's celebrations, to your surprise, there would be a gift with your name. She would sneak out to her secret stash to find something suitable, ensuring no one felt left out.

Like all of us, Betty was frequently reminded that life is swift and uncertain. Just like the grains of sand slipping through an hourglass. Yet, in those moments of uncertainty, it was her unwavering faith and trust in God that sustained her through the pain, loss, guilt, and fog of grief.

Betty gave even when it was difficult, trusting that God would provide. Her heart for others extended beyond her family and church, to rolling pennies for the honor flight, filling boxes for Samaritan's Purse, crocheting hats for newborns, and making homemade cards for the sick and lonely. Giving was by far her love language.

Betty's hourglass of 91 years was surely full, but as the grains of sand became few, she worried she had not been enough. She struggled with the idea of leaving her family, especially Dave. But days before she left this earth, her focus was on eternity, and she verbally prayed for God to take her home.

The family discovered the perfect farewell; surrounding Betty with 72 hours of love, singing, prayer, and reassurance.

As her final moments approached, her last words were 'Stand up, please' as she reached for what they could not see. They lifted her into a tender embrace, and as her body yielded to its final rest, she passed gently from their arms to the arms of her loving savior.

Dave received the last squeeze of her hand. And the hourglass of eternity was reset.

For it was you who formed my inward parts;

you knit me together in my mother's womb.
I praise you, for I am fearfully and wonderfully made.

Wonderful are your works; that I know very well.

My frame was not hidden from you when I was being made in secret,

intricately woven in the depths of the earth.

Your eyes beheld my unformed substance.

In your book were written all the days that were formed for me, when none of them as yet existed.

How weighty to me are your thoughts, O God!

How vast is the sum of them! I try to count them—

they are more than the sand;

I come to the end--I am still with you.

~Psalms 139:13-18 NRS

A Celebration of God's Gift

The shortest verse in the Bible is 'Jesus wept'. He wept at the death of Lazarus and at the sorrow and loss Martha and Mary, Lazarus' sisters felt. Although Jesus was just moments from raising Lazarus from the dead, He still mourned with sorrow.

He taught us two important lessons from this short passage.

First, there is a natural process of mourning. And it is a personal process that each of us must find and experience on our own.

Second Just as God furnished a way out of death for Lazarus by raising him from the dead, He also furnished a way out of death for each of us.

Jesus is the author and chief agent of life - by Jesus' suffering in death, he tasted death for all mankind. Through Jesus' one act of dying, he brought a cancellation of the condemnation of our sins.

Betty knew this, believed it, and trusted God in His word.

I tell you this for two reasons.

First, so you can know that you can have the same assurance Betty had.

The Bible tells us… "for in Adam all die, in Christ all live" Jesus has put death away forever, but it is a gift we must accept.

Second, sickness and death have no authority. Betty is basking in the true light of Jesus. We expect her mansion remodel is already underway, and she is playing all-night cards with her sisters.

For many of you, and especially Dave and the family, your personal sand art has been changed forever. Life will never be quite the same. Do not mourn the grains of sand that have slipped away, but instead, rejoice in the sweet memories, the lessons learned, and the love that will forever linger in your hearts.

Sand Ceremony:

Someone once said if you add your loved one's ashes to an hourglass, they can continue to be part of game night forever. I think Betty would love that.

Of course, the hourglass gift you will receive at the reception does not include Betty's ashes, but they serve as a reminder that life is fleeting, and we have no promise of tomorrow.

Love the people God has given you or who He sets in your path, they are a piece of your sand art, embrace each moment, cherish every connection, live with purpose and gratitude, and do not wait to accept the beautiful gift of eternal life, the time is now.

Dear God, thank you for the gift of life and the beautiful sand art you have given each of us. We are grateful for the hope of salvation that only you can provide. We thank you for Betty, whose presence enriched our lives and whose love, life, and laughter will continue to echo through our hearts.

As the sands of our lives have forever shifted with her passing, we ask for your guidance and comfort for her family and friends; help them find strength and peace as they navigate this new normal.

The Sand Ceremony

What it is: A sand art created during the celebration of life. The sand represents the abundant moments of a person's life. Moments that we touch and are touched by others. This ceremony can include only immediate loved ones or all attendees.

Supplies: Sand art vessel, sand in assorted colors, a funnel, and individual sand containers (optional). Note: If the sand art will be displayed after the ceremony, use colors that will complement the room décor.

Ceremony: As our lives touch, they can never be untouched. Even in fleeting moments, like a grain of sand, whether we are aware or not, we are forever touching each other's lives—sometimes with tiny deeds and other times with significant impact.

We don't always know why something we said or did touched someone's heart, but sometimes we are in the right place at the right time, and we bless, or are blessed by, one another.

The sand represents the people touched or touched by [add name].

As family, friends, and loved ones fill the vessel with sand, it symbolizes the small acts of kindness, friendship, special moments, and love that shape lifetime relationships. Once combined, the grains form an inseparable bond, illustrating the lasting impact on each other's lives.

We used the sand ceremony for Mom's celebration of Life. White sand was already in the bottom of the sand art vessel representing Mom. Dad, my siblings, and I added to the vessel during the ceremony.

After the ceremony, the grandchildren carried the sand art out and they added sand during the reception.

Other family and friends were then invited to add sand to complete the sand art.

We found small containers that were prefilled with an assortment of colors of sand. Each guest received one that they added to the sand art. This ensured that similar amounts of assorted colors were added to create a beautiful rainbow of Mom's life.

Sand art represents the many moments of Mom's life and the many lives Mom touched.

Thank You

I shed countless tears of heartache, joy, regret, and gratitude as I shared these words. It was therapeutic for me, and I thank you for reading.

I hope my story helps you, in some small way as you travel a similar journey with a loved one you adore.

Although this book is written from my heart and perspective, it is important to understand that my siblings and niece did so much more than I did. They stood in the gap, lovingly sacrificing a portion of their lives to do for our mother what she did for us and so many others throughout her lifetime.

Laura, Doreen, Jeannine, Bill, and Jennifer, I know I have already said it, but I am truly proud of us as a family. We are who we are because of the love of our faithful and committed parents. We are better because we walked this journey together. Thank you—I admire and adore you.

And to my father, whose love and dedication to my mother through every change and frustration served as an amazing example of committed love and the true meaning of marriage—thank you, Dad. I love you dearly.

Dianne

References

Barbara Karnes, RN - Gone From My Sight, The Dying Experience, BK Books, Inc. (2012)

Barbara Karnes, RN - The Eleventh Hour, A Caring Guide for the Hours to Minutes Before Death, BK Books, Inc. (2012)

Barbara Karnes, RN – A Time To Live, Living with a Live Threatening Illness, BK Books, Inc. (2012)

Barbara Karnes, RN – Pain At End Of Life, What You Need to Know About End of Life Comfort and Pain Management, BK Books, Inc. (2012)

Barbara Karnes, RN – My Friend I Care, The Grief Experience, BK Books, Inc. (2012)

Julie. Welcome to Hospice Nurse Julie! YouTube, uploaded by Hospice Nurse Julie, 22 May 2023, https://youtu.be/c36_A-giSS4

To be notified of additional writings by Dianne, please join the mailing list using the link below.

JOIN - Dianne's Email List

If you like what you read, a review on Kindle or Amazon would mean the world to me.

About the Author

Dianne is a dedicated life coach and Gallup-certified strengths coach with over 30 years of experience in people and leadership development. Her career has been marked by a profound commitment to helping individuals harness their strengths and achieve their full potential.

In addition to her professional experience, Dianne has devoted 18+ years to caring for the elderly, a journey that has deeply enriched her understanding of compassion, resilience, and the human spirit.

Reflecting on her caregiving experience, she shares, "As a personal caregiver, I have had the pleasure of meeting and working with many charming, seasoned individuals. Behind their lined faces and sometimes puzzled eyes are the lessons and memories of a lifetime. Unlike their family and friends, I did not know them in their prime. I arrived late on the scene, in the remaining moments of the final act. I seldom experience their amazing talents, ability to juggle a family and home-based business, their patience and passion for teaching, sports, young people, or volunteer work; but what I do experience is priceless."

Dianne cared for many seasoned adults, including her close friend Marie—a stranger who became a dear friend over four years—Connie, who faced the relentless challenges of dementia for ten years, and several other wise and prized individuals.

Dianne has spent over 40 years discovering what it means to be a disciple of Christ, growing to understand that Jesus does not expect perfection. Known for her 20-second hugs, she regularly prays that God would use her smile and open arms to share His message of love and hope.

Dianne has shared a 27-year journey with her husband Kelly, during which they planted a church and established a Christian wedding ceremony ministry. Although they ran a church weekly for 10 years, their real ministry has been helping the unchurched add God to the highs and lows of life through weddings, funerals, and baby dedications. They have shared God's love with over four hundred couples and their families. For many, Kelly and Dianne were their only introduction to God. These same couples turned to Kelly and Dianne to celebrate or mourn milestones such as the birth of a baby or the loss of a loved one.

Dianne's unique blend of professional expertise, personal caregiving experience, and spiritual insight provides her with a rich perspective on the challenges and rewards of caregiving, which she passionately shares to inspire and support others on similar journeys.